With God for Caregivers

PRAYERS FOR PEOPLE WHO CARE FOR OTHERS

BRUCE & BECKY DUROST FISH

DIMENSIONS
FOR LIVING
NASHVILLE

A MOMENT WITH GOD FOR CAREGIVERS: PRAYERS FOR PEOPLE WHO CARE FOR OTHERS
Bruce and Becky Durost Fish

Copyright © 1998 by Dimensions for Living

All rights reserved.

No part of this work may be reproduced or transmitted in any form or by any means, electronic or mechanical, including photocopying and recording, or by any information storage or retrieval system, except as may be expressly permitted by the 1976 Copyright Act or in writing from the publisher. Requests for permission should be addressed to Dimensions for Living, 201 Eighth Avenue South, P.O. Box 801, Nashville, TN 37202.

This book is printed on acid-free, recycled, elemental-chlorine-free paper.

Library of Congress Cataloging-in-Publication Data

Fish, Bruce.
  A moment with God for caregivers / Bruce and Becky Durost Fish.
    p.   cm.
  ISBN 0-687-07720-6 (pbk. : alk. paper)
  1. Caregivers—Prayer-books and devotions—English. 2. Caring—Religious aspects—Christianity.   I. Fish, Becky Durost.
II. Title.
BV4910.F57   1998
242'.8—dc21   97-37857

Unless otherwise noted, all Scripture quotations are taken from the *Holy Bible: New International Version*®. Copyright © 1973, 1978, 1984 by the International Bible Society. Used by permission of Zondervan Bible Publishers. All rights reserved.

That noted KJV is from the King James Version of the Bible.

98 99 00 01 02 03 04 05 06 07 — 10 9 8 7 6 5 4 3 2 1

MANUFACTURED IN THE UNITED STATES OF AMERICA

CONTENTS

HIS DIVINE POWER

    The Whisper of Omnipotence 7

    Motivated by Love 8

    Let There Be Light 9

    Night Terrors 10

    Night Songs 11

    Just One More Question 12

    Discerning What Is Best 13

    All Things Laid Bare 14

    Reaching to Heaven 15

    Waiting for God's Time 16

EVERYTHING WE NEED FOR LIFE AND GODLINESS

    Making Adjustments 17

    Time for Myself 18

    When I Am Alone 19

Thanks for God's Grace 20

When Criticized 21

A Timely Word 22

Time for Others 23

When I Need Rest 24

Place of Refuge 25

Our Victory 26

OUR KNOWLEDGE OF THE GOD WHO CALLED US

Holy Ground 27

Attitude Is Everything 28

Trial by Fire 29

Leap of Faith? 30

Weeding the Kingdom 31

Draw Near the Fire 32

Grey Eagle Rising 33

GOD'S GREAT AND PRECIOUS PROMISES

A New Situation 34

Bug Control 35

The End of Exile 36

Good News, Bad News 37

When Money Is Needed 38

Spirit of '76 39

Antidote for Fear 40

The Last Enemy 41

No More Tears 42

Leaving Home 43

YOU MAY PARTICIPATE IN THE DIVINE NATURE

When Feeling the Heat 44

Unbind Him! 45

What Am I Doing for You? 46

New Friends 47

Sorrows of a Servant 48

Foot Care 49

Prayer at Sunset 50

In Good Company 51

Feed My Sheep 52
A Time for Release 53

YOU MAY ESCAPE THE CORRUPTION IN THE WORLD

Guard Duty 54
Misplaced Independence 55
Loving Confrontation 56
When Exhausted 57
Waiting Quietly 58
Becoming an Advocate 59
Anxiety Attacks 60
The One Who Remembers 61
Light in the Darkness 62
Shaped by Choices 63
Idol Thoughts 64

THE WHISPER OF OMNIPOTENCE

*Then a great and powerful wind tore the mountains apart ... but the L*ORD *was not in the wind. After the wind there was an earthquake, but the L*ORD *was not in the earthquake. After the earthquake came a fire, but the L*ORD *was not in the fire. And after the fire came a gentle whisper. When Elijah heard it, he pulled his cloak over his face and went out and stood at the mouth of the cave.*

—*1 Kings 19:11b-13*

Father, we long for a spectacular display of your power. We want to know that you are grappling with the things that threaten our loved ones and us. But although spectacular displays make us feel good for a while, they don't bring peace to our souls. What Elijah needed, what he sought, was a personal word from you. Not the wind, not the earthquake, not the fire, but the gentle whisper. Today, may we hear your whisper of omnipotence and find peace for our souls.

MOTIVATED BY LOVE

We continually remember before our God and Father your work produced by faith, your labor prompted by love, and your endurance inspired by hope in our Lord Jesus Christ.
—*1 Thessalonians 1:3*

Lord, my caregiving in part grows out of my faith, my sense of how you have instructed us to care for our families. But on those tough days when my nose is being rubbed into the worst aspects of servanthood, may my labors also be prompted by love, and may the promise of what you are doing in my life through Christ's work on the cross motivate me to endure.

LET THERE BE LIGHT

God said, "Let there be light," and there was light. God saw that the light was good, and he separated the light from the darkness.
—*Genesis 1:3-4*

Father, light was your chosen tool for fashioning the world. You did not destroy darkness, but gave us a way to understand it. You gave shape to what was formless and drew life out of empty shadow.

Our relationships with those we care for are like that original formless void. We are in a place where we cannot see clearly, and what we dimly perceive frightens us. May your power and presence illuminate us and our loved ones as we care for them. With the help of your creative presence, may we discover a new life and legacy of hope for those we love.

NIGHT TERRORS

He will cover you with his feathers, / and under his wings you will find refuge.... / You will not fear the terror of night, / nor the arrow that flies by day.

—*Psalm 91:4, 5*

Lord, the phone rang at two o'clock this morning. Mom was calling, terrified. Some of this fear is physiologically caused, and the doctor is changing her medication to help alleviate her distress. But some of her fear is not simply a case of chemical imbalances in her body. There is a genuine fear of being alone, of being vulnerable, of feeling life slip away. Be with my mother this night. Cover her with your wings, and may she find refuge in your love.

NIGHT SONGS

By day the LORD directs his love, / at night his song is with me.

—*Psalm 42:8*

Lord, tonight Mom had an asthma attack and it took the better part of an hour to get her breathing comfortably again. She was understandably upset. To help her relax so she could drift back to sleep, we played Mozart's *Eine kleine Nachtmusik* (A Little Night Music). As she nodded off with a slight smile on her face, I thought of how hearing music in the darkness can bring comfort and security. Thank you that no matter how dark the nights of my life may be, your song never ceases.

JUST ONE MORE QUESTION ...

"Where were you when I laid the earth's foundation? / Tell me, if you understand."
—Job 38:4

Father, we watch the mounting losses of our loved ones and feel our own lives slipping away. Their growing dependency haunts us. How can we feel safe when such things happen to those around us?

We are shocked by your response to Job. He asks for an explanation of his suffering and you tell him to reflect on your sovereign power. Is there another lesson for us to learn?

Does your presence in a fallen world sow the seeds of both our suffering and our salvation? And where does comfort come from? When a flood of suffering threatens to carry us away, can we escape by piling up answers around us like sandbags?

Help us remember that what you do not prevent, you still have the power to redeem. May we find you powerfully near to us, as you were to Job when you asked him your thundering questions.

DISCERNING WHAT IS BEST

And this is my prayer: that your love may abound more and more in knowledge and depth of insight, so that you may be able to discern what is best.
—*Philippians 1:9-10*

Lord, it is so difficult to know what is best in this situation. Would activities at the senior center be helpful or harmful? Whom should we hire to supplement our caregiving? Do the social benefits of the foot-care clinic outweigh the difficulties of getting Mom up earlier than she likes?

May we see Mom clearly—have insight into her needs—and be better able to discern what is best.

ALL THINGS LAID BARE

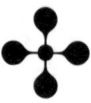

For the word of God is living and active. Sharper than any double-edged sword, it penetrates even to dividing soul and spirit, joints and marrow; it judges the thoughts and attitudes of the heart. Nothing in all creation is hidden from God's sight.
—Hebrews 4:12-13a

Father, give us the courage to manage the truth as you uncover it. May we find it gentle when dealing with the broken places of our lives and immensely strong when confronting our proud ignorance.

Help us to see the truth about those in our care. May our clear vision give them comfort as their understanding fades. Stand with us as we face with them the anguish of lifelong fears and bad habits. Guard their souls from these enemies. Embrace us with your immense love, which always waits for us at the center of every truth that comes from you. Show us the inexhaustible hope that flows from your truth, as we walk together through difficult times. May we, and those we care for, be changed by this encounter.

REACHING TO HEAVEN

Even to your old age and gray hairs / I am he, I am he who will sustain you. / I have made you and I will carry you.

—Isaiah 46:4

Lord, it's fall. A cool breeze nips the air, warning of winter's approach. The leaves are dropping from the trees, and the Canada geese form huge *V*s in the sky, pointing south. Yet as summer's flowers turn brown, and trees stand with bare arms reaching toward heaven, I am still surrounded by beauty: orange mountain ash berries suspended from their branches, streaks of yellow-orange vine maple climbing across the foothills, huge flocks of evening grosbeaks gathered at the feeder. As my loved one prepares for the winter of her life, bare arms reaching toward heaven, may I also see the beauty that marks this season of her life and praise you.

WAITING FOR GOD'S TIME

But I trust in you, O LORD; / I say, "You are my God." / My times are in your hands; / deliver me from my enemies / and from those who pursue me.
—Psalm 31:14-15

Lord, I talked with the receptionist at the eye doctor's. Her father has cancer and has been dying for two years. He's said his good-byes to everyone who knows him. There are no unresolved situations. He is wasting away. The whole family senses that it is his time to go. Yet he remains.

I understand her suffering. The hours of our days are in your hands, but sometimes we question why the last minutes and seconds are necessary. Give me and the others who are caring for my loved one the wisdom to do everything we can to ease her discomfort, and help us trust you with the timing of her departure.

MAKING ADJUSTMENTS

The prudent see danger and take refuge, / but the simple keep going and suffer for it.
—*Proverbs 27:12*

Lord, whenever I face change, some familiar things must also be eliminated from my life. I have added both the hours it takes to care for my parent and the time I need for replenishment. Much as I want to hang onto all my old activities, I can't continue like this.

I need to discern which activities are best put aside during this time of added commitments. Help me to determine which people are most important in my life and then select the activities that will build those relationships and allow my soul to be nurtured. Give me the will to restore balance to my days, and grant me your peace in the choices I make.

TIME FOR MYSELF

Martha was distracted by all the preparations that had to be made. She came to [Jesus] and asked, "Lord, don't you care that my sister has left me to do the work by myself? Tell her to help me!"

"Martha, Martha," the Lord answered, "you are worried and upset about many things, but only one thing is needed. Mary has chosen what is better, and it will not be taken away from her."
—Luke 10:40-42

Lord, there are so many responsibilities in my life. Like Martha, I can only see the needs of other people and what I must do to meet them. Whether I am at home, at work, or at church, people ask things of me, and I feel obligated to say yes. Open my eyes so that, like Mary, I will recognize my own needs not as an expression of selfishness, but as something you honor and are willing to meet—if only I will let some things go and sit at your feet.

WHEN I AM ALONE

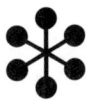

Even though I walk / through the valley of the shadow of death, / I will fear no evil, / for you are with me; / your rod and your staff, / they comfort me.

—*Psalm 23:4*

Lord, I know that there are thousands of caregivers out there, but my friends aren't among them. Their parents are active and healthy. They give me blank stares when I try to describe some middle-of-the-night crisis. They try to be helpful by suggesting activities that my parent can no longer enjoy or do safely. They cannot comprehend how much energy it takes to care for the one who used to care for me. There are days—weeks—when I feel very alone in this situation. Remind me that you are with me as I walk in the shadow of death.

THANKS FOR GOD'S GRACE

The LORD will guide you always; / he will satisfy your needs in a sun-scorched land / and will strengthen your frame.
—Isaiah 58:11

Lord, today went well. There were no new problems—or old problems, for that matter. The sun was shining. Everything worked the way it's supposed to. There were no long waits at traffic lights, no complaints about meals, no objections to taking medicine. Nobody fought. The family smiled. Life was good.

It's so easy to focus on the problems and difficulties that life brings. But today was kissed with a double measure of your grace. Thank you for this break from the ordinary that we all so desperately needed.

WHEN CRITICIZED

O LORD, you have seen this; be not silent. / Do not be far from me, O Lord. / Awake, and rise to my defense! / Contend for me, my God and Lord.
—Psalm 35:22-23

Lord, I just learned that someone was criticizing me behind my back for how I'm taking care of my parent. This person doesn't know the situation. She doesn't know how many professionals I have both advising me about the best care and stopping in to supplement what I'm doing. She never bothered to ask me. Instead she jumped to conclusions and spread lies. I'm angry and hurt and discouraged. Tomorrow I will call her and try to clarify the situation. But tonight I need a defender. I need to know that you will stand up for me.

A TIMELY WORD

A word aptly spoken / is like apples of gold in settings of silver.
—*Proverbs 25:11*

Lord, one of the home healthcare nurses took me aside today and told me how impressed she is by the care we are giving Mom. Thank you for bringing someone into my life who encourages and affirms me. It means so much to have a professional who knows our situation tell me that I'm doing something right.

Help me to remember these words of praise so that when I am criticized by people who don't know the particulars of our situation, I will not take their words to heart. And give me opportunities to pass on this gift of praise to others who cross my path.

TIME FOR OTHERS

Be very careful, then, how you live—not as unwise but as wise.
—*Ephesians 5:15*

Lord, the special needs of my loved one can sometimes block from view the needs of the rest of my family. Yet before I became a caregiver, I made commitments to my spouse, my children. They will be with me long after the need for my caregiving is past. Give me the wisdom to balance my time and attention so that I will not inadvertently sow seeds of bitterness and resentment in the souls of those I love so much.

WHEN I NEED REST

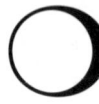

Six days you shall labor and do all your work, but the seventh day is a Sabbath to the LORD your God. On it you shall not do any work.
—*Exodus 20:9-10*

Lord, sometimes it's hard to trust that others will take care of my parents as well as I would. I feel so responsible for them that I want to control every minute of their lives. I want to be there if there's a problem, and I want to be there to prevent any problem from occurring. Give me the faith to trust you with my parents. Then, having released them to you, may I let others participate in my parents' care so that I am free to obey your commands about rest.

PLACE OF REFUGE

He who dwells in the shelter of the Most High / will rest in the shadow of the Almighty. / I will say of the LORD, "He is my refuge and my fortress, / my God, in whom I trust."
—*Psalm 91:1-2*

Father, she sits in her chair, staring out the window, unable to believe in her own life. She is impoverished in the midst of wealth, lonely among friends. Increasingly she feels only her own pain, sees only her own tears, hears nothing but the quiet sounds of death creeping closer. She can find no place of refuge, no shelter from her own fears, no fortress to defend her from the disease that is stealing her sanity.

On some level, she still believes in you, but she trusts no one. A listless, despairing depression stalks her, and she can no longer find her way to you for shelter. Seek her out as she stumbles down this narrowing path, and be a refuge for her tired soul.

OUR VICTORY

"Where, O death, is your victory? / Where, O death, is your sting?" / The sting of death is sin, and the power of sin is the law. But thanks be to God! He gives us the victory through our Lord Jesus Christ.

—*1 Corinthians 15:55-57*

Lord, I saw a side of Mom today that I never thought I'd see again this side of heaven. She had an extra measure of energy, and her mind was sharper than it's been in years. She regaled us with stories and wrote notes to friends. Yesterday she didn't have the strength to sign her name. As I watched her, I wept. The immensity of what I am losing overwhelmed me. But I also felt joy as I haven't in weeks. Something I thought had been lost to me forever was for a brief moment returned, and I was reminded that death will not be the final statement in her life. Thank you for this gift.

HOLY GROUND

Therefore, brothers, since we have confidence to enter the Most Holy Place by the blood of Jesus, ... let us draw near to God with a sincere heart in full assurance of faith.
—*Hebrews 10:19, 22*

Lord Jesus, she stands quietly by the bed of her dying husband, fear held at bay by faith and love. After fifty years, no words are necessary, so she feeds him chips of ice and strokes his fevered face. They both see death's curtain dropping slowly between them. Their eyes embrace, speaking volumes.

I watch the miracle of your love in my mother's eyes, healing my father's soul even as his body is consumed. Those pieces of ice become for them a final communion, offering a promise of new life.

We stand together on holy ground, where life endures in the face of death, and hope has the final word. When my time comes, or my wife's, may we have this kind of confidence and hope, to enter the holy place and do good deeds of love.

ATTITUDE IS EVERYTHING

Your attitude should be the same as that of Christ Jesus: Who, being in very nature God / ... made himself nothing, / taking the very nature of a servant.
—*Philippians 2:5-7*

Father, I admire humility and servanthood, but I don't trust them. They look too much like traps, a standing invitation to every spiritual bully to come and abuse me. And the one who frightens me most is my mother. She can make me feel guilty or sad or inadequate with just a look or a word. Still, you ask me to care for her as Jesus would. He didn't invite or tolerate abuse. He stayed focused on his mission, even when he was acting as a servant. He steadfastly followed the path to the cross, but chose the time of his sacrifice carefully. He even made betrayal a servant of the gospel. He knew that humility without vision is dangerous and that every servant needs a safe path to follow.

Give me a vision for my service to Mom that is powerful enough to break through the roadblocks thrown up by her diseased mind. Help me to take up my cross and follow Jesus.

TRIAL BY FIRE

Shadrach, Meshach and Abednego replied to the king, "O Nebuchadnezzar, ... If we are thrown into the blazing furnace, the God we serve is able to save us from it.... But even if he does not, ... we will not serve your gods or worship the image of gold you have set up."
—Daniel 3:16-18

Father, we live in a world of furnaces. Those who would bind us and cast us in are often people we love. The risk of burning is especially great with those who depend on us for their care. Their needs, desires, demands, and fears bind us. Fiery encounters with them threaten to shrivel our lives, until only ashes remain.

False gods entice us, offering a way of escape. Some ask us to deny the reality of our situation, embracing false hopes and putting off necessary decisions. Others tell us to avoid contact with those who suffer. The most subtle ask us to callously take over the lives of our loved ones, "for their own good." Deliver us from these false gods and from the furnace.

LEAP OF FAITH?

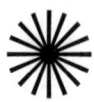

"If you are the Son of God," [the devil] said, "throw yourself down from here. For it is written: 'He will command his angels concerning you / to guard you carefully; / they will lift you up in their hands, / so that you will not strike your foot against a stone.'"

Jesus answered, "It says: 'Do not put the Lord your God to the test.'"

—Luke 4:9-12

Father, is it faith that compels us to continue caring for my mother, or is the devil tempting us to destroy ourselves? Are there precautions we are not taking that we should be? Are there others whom we should be asking to join us in this task? When does faith become presumption?

Tonight I felt myself falling from the precipice, saw the ground rushing toward me. My wife and I need help. We can't go on spending several hours a day, seven days a week with my mom. Save us from this destructive leap of faith. Show us new resources for our battle to keep her living in her home.

WEEDING THE KINGDOM

Jesus told them another parable: "The kingdom of heaven is like a man who sowed good seed in his field. But while everyone was sleeping, his enemy came and sowed weeds among the wheat....

"The servants asked him, 'Do you want us to go and pull them up?'

"'No,' he answered, 'because while you are pulling the weeds, you may root up the wheat with them. Let both grow together until the harvest.'"
—Matthew 13:24-25, 28-30

Father, I want to pull out all the weeds. It frustrates me when you insist on letting them grow. You say you're just raising a good crop for your Kingdom. I'm not so sure. I hate these invaders, these unavoidable expressions of suffering and evil. They shake my faith in your goodness.

The burden of my mother's suffering is a weed, and you have chosen to let it grow. I'm frightened of this weed. Its deep and spreading roots are choking me. I'm dying with her. Protect me and show me how to relieve her suffering. Lord Jesus, help me to build your Kingdom.

DRAW NEAR THE FIRE

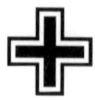

Let us then approach the throne of grace with confidence, so that we may receive mercy and find grace to help us in our time of need.
—Hebrews 4:16

Lord Jesus, you offer us a warm welcome at the throne of grace, but there we also meet the one of whom the Old Testament says, "Our God is a consuming Fire."

Still, you bid us to draw near that fire with its dancing life. You promise us healing and strength in the warmth of your Father's embrace. He burns away the coldness of our hearts and gives them back beating and healthy. As the fire grows within, it transforms us into your likeness.

From the secret places of our lives, you look out with burning compassion on those dependent on our care. Help us pass on to them the gifts received from you, as we bid them to draw near the fire.

GREY EAGLE RISING

Even youths grow tired and weary, / and young men stumble and fall; / but those who hope in the LORD / will renew their strength. / They will soar on wings like eagles; / they will run and not grow weary, / they will walk and not be faint.
—*Isaiah 40:30-31*

Lord, teach me to soar on eagle wings of promise, stronger than my best deeds. Carry me rejoicing into the future, strong with hope.

A NEW SITUATION

If any of you lacks wisdom, he should ask God, who gives generously to all without finding fault, and it will be given to him.

—*James 1:5*

Lord, change is in the air. I'm becoming the primary caregiver for my parent. As much as I think I know what to expect, I know from other experiences that I never can fully comprehend what a change will bring until I've gone through it. I am excited, nervous, and fearful all at once.

As I take on this responsibility, I pray for wisdom and patience. Give me the ability to see situations clearly and to respond rather than react. Give me an understanding mind so that I can provide quality care, and an understanding heart so that the care I give will be filled with compassion. And may I never forget that in every situation, you are with me.

BUG CONTROL

"I will repay you for the years the locusts have eaten.... / You will have plenty to eat, until you are full, / and you will praise the name of the LORD your God, / who has worked wonders for you."

—*Joel 2:25-26*

Lord, Mom is bewildered by all the changes. It's obvious that her need for supervision and care is going to increase in the next few years.

Our lives are being swallowed by her demands and needs, just as surely as if a biblical plague of locusts had appeared. Years from now, who will give us back our lives? Who will restore the years the locusts have eaten?

In the coming days, help us learn to trust in your wisdom, power, and mercy. For if you restore prosperity and hope after judgment, how much more will you do so after tragedy.

THE END OF EXILE

"When seventy years are completed for Babylon, I will come to you and fulfill my gracious promise to bring you back to this place. For I know the plans I have for you," declares the LORD, "plans to prosper you and not to harm you, plans to give you hope and a future."
—Jeremiah 29:10-11

Lord, today Mom sat down at the piano and began to play for the first time in ten years. While others were still listening, I crept off to the kitchen and wept for joy. And through those tears, I glimpsed a future full of hope, for all of us.

Thank you for the joy that slips up on me suddenly; may I appreciate its wonder. Left to myself, grief comes too easily and stays for too long. In the midst of the hard task you have set before me, may I remember that you still have plans, as you did for Israel, to give me a prosperous future full of hope.

GOOD NEWS, BAD NEWS

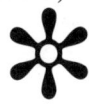

The LORD is my shepherd, I shall not be in want. / He makes me lie down in green pastures, / he leads me beside quiet waters, / he restores my soul. / He guides me in paths of righteousness / for his name's sake.

—Psalm 23:1-3

Father, if it's all the same to you, I'd rather not be a sheep. Sheep are slow and stupid and heedless. They can't survive without supervision. They walk off cliffs, drown while trying to get a drink, and die from eating the wrong thing.

Yet it's not much better being a shepherd, is it? Jesus knew the price of that calling. He said, "I am the good shepherd. The good shepherd lays down his life for the sheep."

Lord, if your Son is willing to be my Shepherd, I'm willing to be his sheep. I'll trust him to restore my soul when I must walk hard paths of righteousness.

WHEN MONEY IS NEEDED

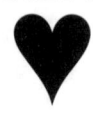

"Do not set your heart on what you will eat or drink;... your Father knows that you need them. But seek his kingdom, and these things will be given to you as well."
—Luke 12:29-31

Lord, I need money. It seems so materialistic to say that, but it's the truth. Our budget was never designed to absorb the costs of caregivers, prescriptions, special diets, and equipment that Medicare and insurance don't cover. Lead me to people who can make me aware of other resources that are available. Give me the courage to admit this problem to the professionals I work with. And most of all, give me the faith to trust that you will provide for our needs.

SPIRIT OF '76

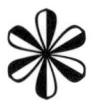

Delight yourself in the LORD / and he will give you the desires of your heart.
—*Psalm 37:4*

Father, childlike delight, that's what I see in Mom's eyes tonight. And I know it came from you.

Last week, she was telling me how much she liked one of her calligraphy pieces, based on the phrase "He Is Risen." She said, "I want to rise like Jesus someday." I swallowed hard and said, "Amen, preach it!"

A few days ago, she was reading the Psalms to me. She talks about all of us getting along by trusting you.

And tonight I see you giving her the desires of her heart. Ten of us who love her are celebrating her seventy-sixth birthday. She's delighted, we're delighted, and I'll bet you're delighted too. May the spirit of this night sustain us all far into the future.

ANTIDOTE FOR FEAR

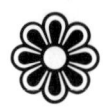

God did not give us a spirit of timidity, but a spirit of power, of love and of a calm, well-balanced and disciplined mind.
—2 Timothy 1:7 (author's paraphrase)

Father, lately we find ourselves calling her "Little Miss Much Afraid," because she reminds us of a character in *Pilgrim's Progress*. She's afraid that children are throwing rocks at her house, even though she lives in a senior development. It's hard to convince her that the noises are coming from the walls themselves, as they heat up and cool down during the day. She's afraid to have anyone looking into her house and keeps the blinds drawn most of the day.

A spirit of timidity and fear is poisoning her life, and we need an antidote soon. She needs your power to stand up to these fears. She needs the assurance of your love to feel safe in the daily routines of life. She needs the calming presence of your mind to stand up against the chaos in her own.

THE LAST ENEMY

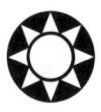

The trumpet will sound, the dead will be raised imperishable, and we will be changed.
—*1 Corinthians 15:52*

Lord, every strategy for dealing with my mother is failing us. An insidious combination of bad choices, mental illness, and dementia is stealing her away. This enemy is too cunning for us. Its immeasurable strength meets us wherever we turn. There is no victory in this world against such a foe.

Teach me to show merciful firmness toward this poor, sick woman. Help me to see past the living death that is consuming her, so I can love the person imprisoned in its grasp. Rescue her soon from this body of death, so she can find a place of wholeness and contentment in your Kingdom. I ask these things in the imperishable and immeasurably strong name of Jesus.

NO MORE TEARS

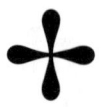

✢

He will wipe every tear from their eyes. There will be no more death or mourning or crying or pain, for the old order of things has passed away."
  —*Revelation 21:4*

Father, she's crying again tonight. Sometimes she cries to get her own way, but these are real tears. I see grief and rage in her eyes; I hear fear and loss in her voice. And I can't do anything to help her.

I can't restore her memory or bring her husband of fifty years back from the grave. I can't bring her old friends, who live hundreds of miles away, any closer. I can't restore her passion for books or music or art. I can't spend every day and all of the nights here to keep loneliness and fear at bay. I can't even promise her that tomorrow will be better; it probably won't. I can't wipe away her tears.

But you can.

I am thankful that we don't have to wait until your Kingdom comes in power to know the reality of your healing presence. Wipe away my mother's tears this night. And while you're at it, could you help me with mine too?

LEAVING HOME

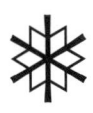

The LORD had said to Abram, "Leave your country, your people and your father's household and go to the land I will show you."
—*Genesis 12:1*

Father, did Abram know what he was getting into when he left home to face the peril and promise of faith?

I didn't. I thought that leaving home was about my choices, but tonight I face a new departure. This time, my home is leaving me. I stand in shocked stillness, on a gray-green hillside. In the distance, I can see the lights of a hospital. There my father's life is slipping away. Sometime tonight he will die. And a part of me goes with him. All his memories of my past life are swallowed up; things I never knew about myself.

I am leaving home again, but what new land of promise opens before me? I must reach for it across the years, must grasp my heritage as a man of faith, a child of Abraham. He would understand.

Lord Jesus, you were also separated from your Father by death. Stand by me this night.

WHEN FEELING THE HEAT

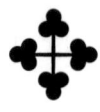

✛

"Blessed is the man who trusts in the LORD, / whose confidence is in him. / He will be like a tree planted by the water / that sends out its roots by the stream. / It does not fear when heat comes.... / It has no worries in a year of drought."
—*Jeremiah 17:7-8*

Lord, this stage of my life feels like a drought. The pressures of caregiving along with the ordinary demands of life sometimes make me think I'm in a desert. Yet you've told us that these times come to everyone. May I place my confidence in your resources rather than in my own strength, and may I draw on your life-giving power every day.

UNBIND HIM!

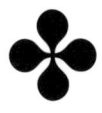

♣

Jesus called in a loud voice, "Lazarus, come out!" The dead man came out, his hands and feet wrapped with strips of linen, and a cloth around his face.

Jesus said to them, "Take off the grave clothes and let him go."

—*John 11:43-44*

Lord Jesus, I am thankful that you let others help when you brought your friend Lazarus back from the dead. It must have surprised these people, who had come to mourn, to find themselves removing his grave clothes.

You still ask us to release people from the things that limit their enjoyment of life. Show us new strategies for freeing those who depend on us for daily care. We can read to those who have lost their sight. We can provide transportation for those who can no longer drive. We can clean a house, or even just a room, for someone who has a crippling disease.

In all our service to those we love, let us remember your command to give them back their lives.

WHAT AM I DOING FOR YOU?

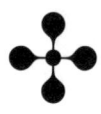

"I tell you the truth, whatever you did for one of the least of these brothers of mine, you did for me."
—Matthew 25:40

Lord, today I heard from a friend who is very successful in her career and very active in our church and community. She wanted me to participate in a church outreach program. You heard the silence when I declined, explaining that taking care of Mom and my family and going to work more than filled my days. She was too polite to ask what others have: "But what are you doing for the Lord?"

Help me to remember that every time I wash Mom's hair, ease her anxieties, or take care of her personal needs, I am doing it for you. Others may not notice, but you see what I am doing and will remember.

NEW FRIENDS

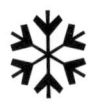

Perfume and incense bring joy to the heart, / and the pleasantness of one's friend springs from his earnest counsel.

—*Proverbs 27:9*

Lord, thank you for bringing new friends into my life, older friends who have walked this road of caregiving before me. It is such a gift to be able to talk with someone who understands the complex issues I'm facing and can make practical suggestions about how to deal with them. In time, may I have the opportunity to do the same for others.

SORROWS OF A SERVANT

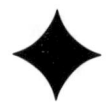

♦

"Now that I, your Lord and Teacher, have washed your feet, you also should wash one another's feet. I have set you an example that you should do as I have done for you."

—*John 13:14-15*

Lord, Mom made an unintentional mess in the bathroom today, but that didn't make it any less disgusting. I cried as I cleaned it up. At times I feel angry with her, and then I feel guilty. How can I be angry at her for actions she can't control?

I'm beginning to realize that much of my anger is an expression of grief. It is hard to watch someone you love deteriorate. If I could legitimately hold her accountable for these accidents, it would mean that she was in better health, that death was farther away. But the truth is I am losing her, and some days the pain is more than I can bear. Give me the courage to face my grief and the grace to serve her in her need.

FOOT CARE

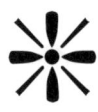

Jesus knew that the Father had put all things under his power, and that he had come from God and was returning to God; so he got up from the meal, took off his outer clothing, and wrapped a towel around his waist. After that, he poured water into a basin and began to wash his disciples' feet, drying them with the towel that was wrapped around him.

—*John 13:3-5*

Lord Jesus, I hate to wash my mother's feet and cut her toenails. Her feet smell because she won't wash them regularly. In her presence, I feel helpless, angry, tired, and desperately sad. Still, I try to help her because I believe you command it.

Lately, an image of you washing the disciples' feet has come to me as I've worked on hers. I see you bending to your task without hesitation, even when you hold the feet of Judas, who you know is about to betray you. Help me to remember who watches over my work and receives it as both a gift and an act of obedience to a command given long ago.

PRAYER AT SUNSET

The heavens declare the glory of God; / the skies proclaim the work of his hands. / Day after day they pour forth speech; / night after night they display knowledge.

—*Psalm 19:1-2*

Lord, today I took a moment to go outside at sunset. The purples and reds and oranges in the west shot across the sky, tinting the clouds in the east with gentle lilacs, pinks, and yellows. As I absorbed the beauty and felt the cool evening breeze brush against my face, the burdens of the day melted away. In that moment, you reminded me how much bigger you are than the situations I face. Thank you that I can rely on you to be with me and help me through whatever challenges I face. Thank you for your strength and for the beauty you created—in the world that surrounds me and in the people for whom I care.

IN GOOD COMPANY

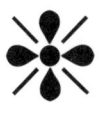

My God, my God, why have you forsaken me?
—*Psalm 22:1*

Father, tonight there is only pain, shock, and rage. She hit my wife, and I'm going to make her pay. I rush into her bedroom. A vision of your Son explodes in my mind, paralyzing me in mid-step, a moment from revenge. He stands silently while they slap him, strip him, whip him, and send him out to hang—nailed to rough wood, all dignity denied. So I embrace my wife instead. All is silent, except for her tears. They fall freely and leave bleeding stripes down my back. Stiff with pain, we stand together, fighting for breath; hanging in a moment of time without end, pierced by the demands of faith and the decaying life of my mother. We thirst for deliverance from her. Is it finished?

Not yet, you seem to say. "I am crucified with Christ: nevertheless I live; yet not I, but Christ liveth in me" (Galatians 2:20 KJV).

FEED MY SHEEP

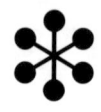

When they had finished eating, Jesus said to Simon Peter, "Simon son of John, do you truly love me more than these?" "Yes, Lord," he said, "you know that I love you." Jesus said, "Feed my lambs."
—*John 21:15*

Father, lately she almost looks like a sheep: the tottering gait, the blank expression from eyes that seem no longer quite human. But her surroundings tell a different story. There are books, thousands of them, on every topic imaginable. Great stacks of sheet music for piano and organ are neatly stored near hundreds of records and tapes. Several pieces of calligraphy, with biblical themes, are the last things she finished before illness narrowed her world.

But today I see need and fear in her great sheep-eyes; not faith, creativity, and the love of beauty. Help me to see past the ravages of disease to that hidden and holy place where a child of yours waits for her release. Give me the strength to feed this lamb until you take her in your arms and carry her to perfection in Jesus.

A TIME FOR RELEASE

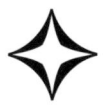

For just as the sufferings of Christ flow over into our lives, so also through Christ our comfort overflows.
—*2 Corinthians 1:5*

Lord, you know what it is like to turn the responsibility for your mother over to another. On the cross, you entrusted John with her care. Now it is my turn, and although it is clear that others must care for my mother, I am filled with grief as I prepare her for this change. Both Mom and I feel so familiar with your sufferings. At this moment, let us overflow with your comfort as well.

GUARD DUTY

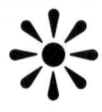

Set a guard over my mouth, O LORD; / keep watch over the door of my lips.

—Psalm 141:3

Lord, on days when I'm tired (and lately that's most days), it's so easy for me to let slip a harsh word, a sarcastic retort, a cutting comment. I concentrate on being careful about what I say when I'm caregiving, and then when I relax with the rest of the family, I say something hurtful to them. I know I need to get more rest, but on those days when rest isn't an option, set a guard over my mouth. Protect my loved ones from my unwitting barbs.

MISPLACED INDEPENDENCE

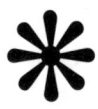

✻

"O Jerusalem, Jerusalem,... how often I have longed to gather your children together, as a hen gathers her chicks under her wings, but you were not willing."
—*Matthew 23:37*

Lord, the man who was once so competent must now rely on others, and he doesn't like it. Can I blame him? I don't think I would like it either. But he puts himself in danger when he climbs up on chairs to get something that's out of reach or refuses to use his cane or snitches the keys and drives when he's not supposed to.

I would love to be able to make him do the right thing, but I can't. You, who have the power to make us obey, in your wisdom allow all your children to make mistakes. Help me to respect his right to make choices—even bad ones—while being mindful of his best interests and the best interests of others. And when he suffers the consequences of his bad choices, keep my lips from saying, "I told you."

LOVING CONFRONTATION

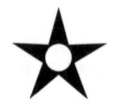

Speaking the truth in love, we will in all things grow up into him who is the Head, that is, Christ.
—*Ephesians 4:15*

Lord, I get scared when I know I need to confront my parents about something. I don't want to set off a verbal nuclear exchange, but I'm beginning to realize that avoiding issues can be just as destructive. Through my silence, I'm telling my parents that it is acceptable for them to use their illness as an excuse for treating me badly. I begin to seethe with anger, and then something happens and I explode.

Help me to deal lovingly, yet firmly, with issues as they come up. Give me the determination to set reasonable limits on their demands. And as I "speak the truth in love," may we all become more like you.

WHEN EXHAUSTED

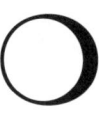

The angel of the LORD came back a second time and touched [Elijah] and said, "Get up and eat, for the journey is too much for you." So he got up and ate and drank. Strengthened by that food, he traveled forty days and forty nights until he reached Horeb, the mountain of God.

—*1 Kings 19:7-8*

Lord, I'm exhausted. I am at the end of my resources. I cannot cope with one more demand, one more sharp word, one more crisis. I am filled with despair. Give me the courage to rest. Help me to act on the knowledge that if I do not take care of myself, I cannot help those you have given into my care. Protect me from false guilt, an unwillingness to let go, fear of what might happen when I'm gone—the chains that imprison me in an unhealthy situation. Restore my body and soul so that I can return to this task filled with joy.

WAITING QUIETLY

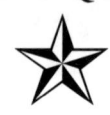

The LORD is good to those whose hope is in him, / to the one who seeks him; / it is good to wait quietly / for the salvation of the LORD.
—Lamentations 3:25-26

Lord, today we sat in the waiting room at the doctor's office for an hour and a half. The doctor had been called away by an emergency. At one point, Mom's eyes twinkled, and she said, "I know how to get their attention. I'll just throw myself down on the floor and scream." I chuckled. Like her, I'm much better at screaming than at waiting quietly. Thank you that when I'm waiting for you, it isn't because someone else is more urgently in need of your attention. You are also waiting—waiting for the fullness of time, that point when everything is completely ready. As I sit in your waiting room, may I put aside my fretfulness and wait quietly, filled with your peace.

BECOMING AN ADVOCATE

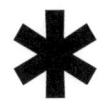

✱

"Be strong and courageous. Do not be terrified; do not be discouraged, for the LORD your God will be with you wherever you go." —Joshua 1:9

Lord, there are days when I feel like nobody takes me seriously. I deal with so many professionals: doctors, home healthcare nurses, physical therapists, social workers, senior advocates—the list never seems to end. When I report something, they say, "We can understand how you'd conclude that, given your perspective." I think what they really mean is, "Your perspective is skewed, so your conclusions are faulty." Sometimes their advice conflicts, and I seem to be an unwilling soldier on a philosophical battleground rather than an important member of a team whose mission is to provide excellent care.

Give me the energy to stand up for my family member, to insist on explanations for why treatments are being continued or changed. When these professionals seem to ignore my input, give me the courage to ask why they think my perceptions are wrong. And let me never forget that you are with me in this situation.

ANXIETY ATTACKS

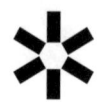

Comfort, comfort my people, / says your God. / Speak tenderly to Jerusalem, / and proclaim to her / that her hard service has been completed.
—Isaiah 40:1-2

Lord, she is afraid. Afraid of pain, of loneliness, of forgetting something or someone important. Earlier in her life she was able to put her fear aside and trust you; now she seems unable to resist its power. She clings to those of us around her, and often her hold brings with it a weight that is more than I can bear. Give me strength. Use me this day to speak words of comfort and reassurance to her. Help me to see the fear behind her anger. And make your presence more real to both of us than any of the fears we face.

THE ONE WHO REMEMBERS

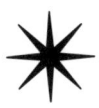

"Can a mother forget the baby at her breast / and have no compassion on the child she has borne? / Though she may forget, / I will not forget you!"
—Isaiah 49:15

Lord, Mom is confused. I often wonder if she knows who I am. It seems incredible that a mother could actually forget the child she gave birth to, but it happens every day. Diseases of the mind and body tear away the ability to recognize friends, spouses, and children. While I grieve the loss of my mother, may I also be comforted in the knowledge that you will never forget me. As I cry out, your arms will continue to enfold me.

LIGHT IN THE DARKNESS

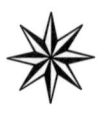

"See, darkness covers the earth / and thick darkness is over the peoples, / but the L<small>ORD</small> rises upon you / and his glory appears over you."
—*Isaiah 60:2*

Lord, today was one of those days when I felt immersed in darkness. We could see new signs of decline in Mom's condition, work went badly, and it was cold and rainy. This darkness is tangible—thick and oppressive. Give me eyes to see your glory rising above the darkness of my situation. Shine your bright light on my path.

SHAPED BY CHOICES

Teach me, O LORD, to follow your decrees; / then I will keep them to the end.
—*Psalm 119:33*

Lord, some of Mom's friends visited today. As I sat listening to these people who've lived seven and eight decades, I was struck by how the pattern of their choices had shaped the outcome of their lives. Those who had chosen to complain for decades are now bitter. Those who had extended themselves to others are now full of joy. May I be aware of the choices I am making today and of the fruit they will bear in the future.

IDOL THOUGHTS

"You shall not make for yourself an idol.... [F]or I, the LORD your God, am a jealous God, punishing the children for the sin of the fathers to the third and fourth generation of those who hate me, but showing love to a thousand generations of those who love me and keep my commandments."
—Exodus 20:4-6

Father, I like my mom's big green overstuffed chair. Still, I'm determined to sell it. To me, it's an ungodly relic. From it, she ruled through tantrums, abuse, and the general fear of her displeasure. She did it to her heart's content and her soul's great loss. Yet I see her soul resting safe with you, cleansed of such corruption.

As I sat in the chair one last time tonight, years of memories floated up quietly, like dust motes in front of a sunny window. Then a cloud of grief covered the sun. Alone in the darkness, I felt the power of the idol stirring, felt the weight of my mother's sin. Lord, help me to sort out the contradictory influences of a parent who loved me imperfectly. May I remember that she was deceived by idols. Help me to follow you to sacred places of comfort and rest.